Low Blood Pressure: Silent Killer

Table of Contents

Introduction

Feeling dizzy or nauseous? Good news! A new member is coming in your family. But what if I tell you the patient is a guy? Confused? Don't be. Not all the time does dizziness or nausea bring the good news of the arrival of a baby; sometimes your body may also warn you like these about your low blood pressure.

Low blood pressure is a health condition which happens in people where the pressure of their blood appears to be abnormally low in their arteries. This can cause many complications, which are mostly not serious but can take a risky turn if not paid attention to. The way your stomach needs a food supply to provide you with energy and nutrients, likewise your brain and heart need a constant supply of oxygen transported by the blood. A low blood pressure will translate to less blood, and therein less oxygen that is delivered to the organs. And when the brain doesn't get enough oxygen this "giddiness" or "lightheadedness" effect takes place where your world is spinning and you feel woozy and nauseous.

Chapter 1- Pressure of Low Blood Pressure

Before you dig down the root of low blood pressure, you should first be acquainted with the basic information – what is blood pressure?

Blood pressure, as the term suggests, refers to the pressure that blood exerts against the walls of the arteries when it is pumped out by the heart. Every time your heart beats, blood is pumped around your body through the arteries. The blood pressure hits the maximum limit when your heart beats and pumps out the blood into the arteries. This pressure is known as "systolic pressure". Naturally, between the beats when the heart is at rest, the blood pressure drops to its minimum level and this pressure is called "diastolic pressure". These two limits are required to determine your blood pressure. Your blood pressure reading is defined as the format systolic/diastolic, for instance, 110/70. In this case, your systolic pressure, or the top value, is 110 while the diastolic pressure, or the minimum value, is 70.

Generally, the blood pressure reading between 90/60 and 140/90 is considered to be normal. Although it varies according to the individual body structure, age, gender and health condition, still blood pressure reading below 90/60 is considered to be low.

Most of the time, people suffer from high blood pressure and, hence, they always try to keep their blood pressure at a minimum level. But extremely low blood pressure can also be proved to be very dangerous for people and can cause serious damage to organs. Low blood pressure means that the organs of the body are getting less amount of blood, and consequently, an insufficient amount of oxygen. Lack of oxygen can temporarily shut down vital organs, like heart and brain, or may even get collapsed and make you go into a coma.

There are cases where people suffer from low blood pressure all the time. They do not face any kind of complications or symptoms and can lead a normal life. The low blood pressure seems to be normal for them and this range becomes optimum for these people. Conversely, people sometimes experience a sudden drop in blood pressure below their normal level and feel uncomfortable. This condition is medically termed as "hypotension".

Low blood pressure, or hypertension, usually happens because of dehydration, blood loss, some antihypertensive medications or certain health conditions. Some may even feel signs of reduced blood pressure when they stand up quickly. Point to be noted is that low blood pressure or hypertension is an issue only if someone faces the symptoms, such as fainting, dizziness, nausea, or in an extreme situation, becomes shocked or suffers from life-threatening consequences.

Mechanism of Blood Pressure Generation

When the heart is relaxed during the state of diastole, blood from the lungs fills the left ventricle from the heart. This ventricle then pumps blood into the arteries by contraction; the state is called systole. During systolic pressure when the ventricles contract, the blood pressure in the artery remains very high as the ventricle pushes the blood in the arteries with force. The pulse that we feel when we push our fingers against an artery is due to the left ventricular contraction that pumps blood into the arteries.

There are two factors that basically determine the blood pressure, those are: i) resistance exerted by the walls of the arterioles, and ii) amount of blood that the left ventricle of the heart pumps into the arteries.

For obvious reason, blood pressure seems to be higher when more blood is pumped into the arteries, or when the arterioles become stiff or narrow. Blood flowing through the narrow passage of arterioles raises the blood pressure. The narrowing of the arterioles occurs due to the contraction of the surrounding muscles. The arterioles of aged patients become narrow or stiff when they suffer from atherosclerosis. On the contrary, blood pressure becomes low if the flow of blood is less, or the width of the arterioles is wider and is more flexible for which the flow of blood faces fewer resistances, and therefore, exerts less pressure on arteriole walls.

Maintenance of Normal Blood Pressure

In normal condition, the body activates several mechanisms to help maintain the optimum blood flow and blood pressure. The mechanisms include sensors that can sense the pressure of blood on artery walls and send signals to the heart, veins, arterioles, kidneys. These body parts then make adjustments to increase or reduce blood pressure until an optimum level is reached.

The body maintains normal blood pressure in several ways by adjusting cardiac output (amount of blood pumped into the arteries by the heart), regulating the amount of blood in veins, the volume of blood and the resistance in the arteries. The necessary adjustments made by heart, veins, arteries and kidneys to regulate blood pressure are:

- **The heart contracts and expands more frequently** – By doing this, the heart can pump blood into the arteries more forcefully and, hence, increase blood pressure due to more blood flow in veins and arteries.

- **The expansion and contraction of veins** – In the case of high blood pressure, veins expand to collect more blood into the veins and, so, heart pumps less blood into the arteries. As a result, blood pressure gets lowered. On the contrary, in the case of hypotension the veins are narrowed to squeeze out as much blood to the heart as possible. The heart then pumps more blood into the arteries and, hence, blood pressure rises.

- **The contraction and expansion of arterioles** – Like the veins, the arterioles also expand and contract to maintain optimum blood pressure. Arterioles expand to reduce blood pressure by creating less resistance, whereas these contracts to resist blood flow more and increase blood pressure.

- **The kidneys regulate blood pressure by increasing or decreasing the quantity of urine production** – Urine is nothing but water that has been excreted out of the blood. When the kidneys secrete out urine, the volume of blood in the veins and arteries reduces which, consequently, reduces blood pressure. On the other hand, when less urine is produced, more blood fills the veins and arteries which ultimately exerting more pressure on the walls of veins and arteries, and elevates the blood pressure. Other mechanisms can regulate blood pressure in seconds while this procedure requires hours and days to affect. For instance, if a severe laceration from an injury occurs, or if stomach ulcers bleed, then this can lower blood pressure. The body quickly responds to increase blood pressure by making appropriate above adjustments, unless the blood flow becomes out of control.

Chapter 2- Know More About Low Blood Pressure

Blood Pressure – How Low Can It Go?

People think that only high blood pressure is dangerous for them, but they remain unaware of the fact that low blood pressure can also become life-threatening, or can even cause death in extreme cases. Although there are only a few records of hypotension patient going into a coma, or dying from stroke out of low blood pressure, still it is better to keep blood pressure at an optimum level. After all, the extreme of anything is never good for anyone. Therefore, it is always a good idea to be well-informed about the risks, symptoms, prevention and cure related to hypotension.

If a range of blood pressure is low for you, it does not mean it will be low for someone else too. It might be normal for them. Chronically low blood pressure in patients is considered to be very low by most doctors only if this causes severe symptoms. According to some experts, blood pressure is considered to be lower than normal when any one of the readings drops, that is, either below 90 mm Hg systolic or below 60 mm Hg diastolic. For example, if your diastolic pressure is perfect 70 but your systolic pressure drops down to 80, then your blood pressure will be counted as lower than optimum pressure.

The sudden downfall in blood pressure levels can be injurious to health. A sudden plunge of only 20 mm Hg from 100 systolic to 80 mm Hg systolic can result in dizziness, vomiting or fainting since your brain gets a shortage of blood and, subsequently, low oxygen to function properly. Sometimes uncontrolled bleeding, allergic reactions or severe infections can result in a huge drop in blood pressure which can cause very serious damage or may even be life-threatening.

Highly active people or athletes regularly carry out exercises. For this, they have slower heart rate and lower blood pressure than those who are not that fit. In a general sense, people who eat healthily, do not smoke and maintain a normal weight tend to have lower blood pressure than others. But in rare cases, sudden fall in blood pressure can also indicate the presence of any life-risking disorder in your body.

Different Types of Blood Pressure

There are different types of low blood pressure or hypotension. People who always suffer from low blood pressure are patients of *chronic asymptomatic hypotension*. Usually, they do not face any kind of signs or symptoms and can lead a normal life without any treatment or medical help. This low blood pressure is actually normal for them.

Other kinds of low blood pressure can be seen when the blood pressure suddenly becomes too low. The symptoms of this abrupt fall vary from mild to extremely severe. This type of hypotension can classify into three categories, these are *orthostatic hypotension, neurally mediated hypotension* and *severe hypotension* related to **shock**.

1. Orthostatic Hypotension – It is the most common type of hypotension that occurs when you stand up from lying or sitting position. That is why you feel light-headed or dizzy, or may even become unconscious.

Generally, whenever you stand up the gravity causes most of your blood to be collected in your legs. Your body makes up for it by raising the heart to beat rate and by constricting the blood vessels to ensure that enough blood reaches the brain. Patients with orthostatic hypotension this mechanism of compensating does not work and so blood pressure falls. As a result, they feel light-headedness, blurred vision, dizziness, or they even faint. This fall in blood pressure only lasts for a couple of seconds or minutes after standing up. That is why in this situation you need to sit or lie down calmly for a while until your blood pressure returns to normal level.

Orthostatic hypotension can occur because of several reasons, such as dehydration, large varicose veins, heart problems, burns, prolonged bed rest, pregnancy, diabetes, excessive heat and certain neurological disorders. Drugs can also be the culprit behind this condition. Some of the examples of such drugs include those that are used to treat hypertension, like diuretics, calcium channel blockers, beta blockers and angiotensin-converting enzyme (ACE) inhibitors, or antidepressants, or even medications that are used to treat erectile dysfunction and Parkinson's disease.

The condition of low blood pressure can occur to people of all ages. However, older people are common victims (around 20% are over 65 years old), or those who are weak or have poor health. Most commonly, this happens to people who stand up suddenly after working for a long time in a crouching position, or were sitting crossing their legs for a while. The treatment of orthostatic hypotension often focuses on underlying health issue as this condition usually happens in the response to other medical complications. Rarely, people suffer from orthostatic hypotension and also hypertension when they lie down.

2. Postprandial hypotension - It is a type of orthostatic hypotension that can result in sudden fall in blood pressure after having a meal. This condition is common among older people. Just like the way blood get collected in your feet when you stand up, a large amount of blood also flows to the digestive system after eating a meal. Normally, the body tries to compensate for this by increasing heart beat rate and by constricting some blood vessels to regulate an optimum blood pressure. But this mechanism fails in patients with postprandial hypotension and so they feel faintness, dizziness or fall down.

Moreover, patients with high blood pressure, or disorder of central nervous system such as Parkinson's disease, are mostly at high risk of developing postprandial hypotension. Consuming low dosage of blood pressure drugs and eating small, low-carbohydrate meals may help to ease symptoms.

3. Neurally Mediated Hypotension – When patients suffer from neurally mediated hypotension (NMH), their blood pressure drops down if they keep standing for a long time. As a result, they feel like vomiting, dizzy, or may even faint. NMH can also happen if you experience the scary, upsetting or unpleasant situation. Mostly children and young adults are affected from neutrally mediated hypotension than other age group people. As they grow, they overcome this condition.

The main reason behind this type of hypotension is the miscommunication between the brain and the heart. Generally, keeping standing for a long time pools the leg with blood which the body tries to counteract by normalizing the blood pressure. Patients with NHM cannot do so; rather the nerves in their heart's left ventricle send the brain a wrong signal that blood pressure is very high and not too low. As a result, the brain reduces heart rate which further decreases the blood pressure and pools more blood in the legs. The brain does not get sufficient amount of blood for which the patient feels dizzy and faints.

4. Multiple System Atrophy with Orthostatic Hypotension – The low blood pressure state in this condition happens because of the damaged nervous system. This rare disorder is also known as "Shy-Drager syndrome" and is caused due to progressive damage to the autonomic nervous system, that controls breathing, blood pressure, heart rate, digestion and other involuntary functions in the body. Although this syndrome can be related to muscle tremors, problems with coordination and speech slowed movement and incontinence, but its chief characteristic is severe orthostatic hypotension along with extremely high blood pressure when lying down.

5. Severe Hypotension Linked to Shock – Shocking is the most dangerous and serious life-threatening health condition where the blood pressure plunges so low that vital organs, such as kidneys, brain, etc., starve of oxygen and as a result cannot function well. Compared to other types of hypotension, the blood pressure drops the lowest in the state of shock. For this, shock can prove to be the most fatal, if left untreated. A lot of things can influence shocks, such as profuse blood loss, severe burns, allergic reactions, serious infections and poisoning. If left untreated, shock can even cause death.

Hypotension or low blood pressure can be found in anyone, although certain age groups and other factors influence the cause of some types of low blood pressure.

o **Age** – Adults older than 65 years are most at risk of experiencing drops in blood pressure after having a meal or after standing for a long time. It has been already mentioned that neutrally mediated hypotension (NMH) occurs due to miscommunication between the heart and the brain. This type of hypotension is primarily seen in younger adults or children.

o **Medicinal drugs** – Patients with high risk of getting low blood pressure are those who are on some particular drugs, such as alpha blockers or other high blood pressure inhibitors.

o **Some diseases** – People with health complications, like diabetes, certain heart conditions, or Parkinson's disease, tend to be prone to get low blood pressure more than the others.

Low blood pressure should not be ignored. Even the moderate range of low blood pressure can make you faint and injured from falling down, and not just feel dizzy or weak. A severe problem with low blood pressure due to any cause or medications can starve your body of oxygen. As a result, your vital organs will not be able to function properly and lack of oxygen will ultimately damage your brain and heart.

The good thing is you do not need to bother yourself with worrisome preparations to check your blood pressure. All you may need to do is to wear something short-sleeved during your appointment so that the doctor can fit the blood pressure cuff properly around your arm. Since appointments to doctors usually do not take much long but there a lot of matters remain to be discussed, so it is always a good idea to prepare your queries prior to your appointment.

Furthermore, many people have the tendency to stop taking medications whenever they start to feel better. Let me remind you, this may result in serious complications in the future for which it may even cause your death! Therefore, do not ever stop taking any prescribed medication that keeps your blood pressure at optimum level without taking advice from your doctor.

What Can You Do Prior to An Appointment?

Preparing yourself for an appointment to the doctor can help you satisfy your queries and make your visit worthwhile. The following bullet points are some guidelines that you can follow as a beginner:

- **Be mindful of any pre-appointment requirements** – When you make the appointments, make sure you ask your doctor whether you need to do anything special, such as drink lots of water for a urine test, or refrain from eating and consuming medicines for a blood test.

- **Make a list of all complications you face** – If you are facing any discomfort or symptoms, even the simplest ones, make a list of those and inform your doctor. What might seem simple to you, may be a signal sent by your body for something serious.

- **Mark down all key professional and personal data** – You should never hide anything from your doctor. Inform him/her without being shy about all the important life changes, family medical history (e.g. low blood pressure), stresses and so on. Some personal matters can also affect your health greatly.

- **Write down all medicines or drugs you are taking** – Inform your doctor about all your vitamins or supplements to avoid reaction with other medicines.

- **Take someone along with you** – It is not always possible to remember everything your doctor says. You can take a family member or a friend with you so that you don't miss out any information given during an appointment. An extra pair of ears is always better than one.

- **Discuss your diet and exercise** – Don't forget to ask your doctor about what your diet (allowed and restricted) and required exercises to keep you healthy.

- **Pen down all questions to ask** – Since your time is limited, you might want to write all your questions to save time from most important ones to least important. You may also as other questions during your talk. Some basic questions for hypotension may include:
  - Why are you having the complications or symptoms?
  - What other cause it might be?
  - What type of test is required?
  - Which treatment is appropriate? Overall cost?
  - Which foods and exercises to adopt or avoid?
  - How often should you be tested?
  - How to best manage all your health issues together?
  - Do you need a specialist or generic alternative to the drug?
  - Any other restrictions to follow?
  - Any brochure or website to follow?

Chapter 3-Low Blood Pressure: How & When

If you have read through the above literature, then you know all about the 'what(s)' of low blood pressure. This chapter is a bit lengthy but is worth reading as it will discuss the causes, symptoms, treatments and other vital information regarding low blood pressure.

Causes of Low Blood Pressure

Let us first start with the identification of all the roots of evil hypotension. A sphygmomanometer is a device by which you can measure your blood pressure. If the reading falls 30 mm Hg below the person's normal blood pressure, then it is considered to be hypotension. Frequent reasons that are responsible for lowering blood pressure include medicines, conditions that decrease the amount of blood pumped by the heart and some agent to make the blood thin. Some of the common factors that can cause low blood pressure are:

➢ Common causes of fainting include fear, insecurity, emotional stress or pain.

➢ Dehydration can thin down the blood volume. In extreme cases, hypovolemic shock can occur which can even result in death within few minutes or hours.

- Body pushing blood into the vessels of the skin as a reaction to heat. This causes dehydration.
- Donation of blood.
- Pregnancy: The mother's circulatory system expands rapidly for which blood pressure drops. This is normal and becomes usual after giving birth.
- Loss of blood due to accident or deep injury.
- Internal bleeding from perforated ulcer of the stomach.
- Fluid loss due to diuretics.
- Medicines for depression, heart disease, or high blood pressure.
- Severe allergy, like anaphylaxis, is caused by food, medicines, latex or insect poison. Apart from hypotension, this allergy can induce breathing problems, hives, itching and a swollen throat.
- Infections like toxic shock syndrome (septicemia) can enter the bloodstream and can cause a drop in blood pressure.
- Nervous system disorder, like Parkinson's disease.
- Endocrine issues: Parathyroid disease, such as Addison's disease where your adrenal glands cannot produce enough hormones to maintain blood pressure. Also, low blood sugar (hypoglycemia) and diabetes can cause hypotension.
- Heart disease: Bradycardia can obstruct the pumping of blood by the heart muscles.

➢ Malnutrition: Lack of nutrients, such as vitamin B-12 and folate, can inhibit the body from producing enough red blood cells (anemia) for which blood pressure can fall.

Some medicines that can result in blood pressure drop are:

- Tadalafil (Cialis) or sildenafil (Viagra), particularly in combination with the heart medication nitroglycerin.
- Diuretics (water pills), such as hydrochlorothiazide (Microzide, Oretic) and furosemide (Lasix).
- Medicines for Parkinson's disease, such as pramipexole (Mirapex) or those containing levodopa.
- Some types of antidepressants (tricyclic antidepressants), including doxepin (Silenor), trimipramine (Surmontil), imipramine (Tofranil) and protriptyline (Vivactil).
- Alpha blockers like labetalol and prazosin (Minipress).
- Beta blockers, like atenolol (Tenormin), timolol and propranolol (Inderal, Innopran XL, others).

Low blood pressure can also happen because of lifestyle choice, age, inherited genes or can also be related to being healthy or active. It is normal for your blood pressure to vary according to the workload you have to deal with. Outside temperature, work stress, and your food habit can all affect your blood pressure reading. This is why it is important to always check the reading in the same condition to maintain consistency. If your blood pressure is still low, then your physician will try to find out the reason behind it:

- **Time of day**: Blood pressure is generally less overnight when you sleep, increases a few hours before you wake up, and continues to increase during the day, reaching its highest during mid-afternoon.

- **Stress or relaxation level**: The more relaxed you are, the lower the blood pressure you'll have.

- **The amount of exercise done**: Initially, exercise will elevate your blood pressure, but if you are healthy and exercise daily, then you'll have hypotension when you'll rest.

- **Outside temperature**: Blood pressure can fall on a warm day.

- **After eating**: When food is about to be digested, your blood is diverted to the gut. Hence, the blood pressure falls elsewhere in your body.

- **Age**: As you get older, the blood pressure generally increases, although it is more common that the reading falls after eating and movement when you age.
- **Genes:** According to some research, hypotension or low blood pressure is genetic. If your parents or family members have this condition, then you'll also get this.

Signs and Symptoms of Low Blood Pressure

If the low blood pressure is natural for someone, then the person hardly faces symptoms. In this case, the person may not even require any treatment. However, low blood pressure can sometimes indicate the fact that not enough blood and oxygen are reaching the brain, heart, and other vital organs. Hence, some underlying health complications exist that are creating all the signs and symptoms to warn us:

- ❖ Lightheadedness or dizziness
- ❖ Unsteadiness
- ❖ Fainting (syncope)
- ❖ Distraction/Lack of concentration
- ❖ Blurred vision
- ❖ Nausea or vomiting
- ❖ Clammy, cold, pale skin
- ❖ Shallow, rapid, breathing

- Palpitation (sudden rapid and noticeable heart beats)
- Feeling fatigue or weak
- Depression and Stress
- Feeling confusion
- Abnormal thirst

The above-mentioned symptoms are generally of orthostatic hypotension and neurally mediated hypotension (NMH). Orthostatic hypotension happens within a very short time, few seconds or minutes after you stand up from sitting or lying position. These patients feel that they are about to faint, or they may actually faint. In this case, to overcome the signs and symptoms they should sit or, even better, lie down for a while until the blood pressure returns to normal level. Likewise, the signs and symptoms of neutrally mediated hypotension occur in response to the scary, upsetting or unpleasant situation, or if you keep standing for a long time. The fall in blood pressure with neurally mediated hypotension do not last for a long time and easily goes away if you sit or lie down for a while with your eyes closed until you feel normal.

Even for severe low blood pressure which ends up in shock, the above-enlisted symptoms are included with some additional abrupt effects.

In the state of shock, sufficient blood and oxygen do not reach the brain, heart and other vital organs of the body. Dizziness, light-headedness, confusion, and sleepiness are some of the early signs and symptoms indicating that the brain is being deprived of enough oxygen and blood flow.

During the earliest stages of shock, the signs or symptoms are hardly noticeable and are very difficult to detect. For aged people, the primary sign can be confusion. As time passes, the state of shock also gets worse, until a time comes when the person cannot even sit straight up without feeling dizzy and passing out. If this state of shock continues, then the person will become unconscious. In the worst case scenario, if the condition of shock is not treated right away then this may even lead to fatal consequences.

Depending on the root cause of shock, other signs and symptoms may vary. If the state of shock is caused by major loss of blood volume from an accident or illness, or is induced from the poor pumping action of heart due to heart failure, then the following signs and symptoms may happen:

- Often the skin color becomes pale or blue. The patient may also have cold and sweaty hands and skin. When you press the skin, the color and the depth returns to normal very slowly than the usual time. In addition, a bluish network of veins may appear under the skin.

- The pulse rate becomes more rapid and weaker.
- The patient tends to take short and very rapid breaths.

When the blood vessels relax extremely, this may result in shock, such as "vasodilatory shock". This is the state when a person feels flushed and warm at the beginning. After a while, the person's skin becomes sweaty and cold and, eventually, the patient feels very tired and sleepy. Shock is not normal, rather an emergency. This must be treated without any delay. If a person faces the signs and symptoms of shock, then he or she must call the emergency number for assistance.

Chapter 4- Be Deterrent, Analyse and Treat It Well

Before jumping into any conclusion, the first and foremost task must be to properly diagnose the main reason or underlying health issue that is causing all the signs and symptoms of low blood pressure. In this case, your doctor will prescribe you some tests or procedures to identify the main culprit behind. Only after this, proper treatment and medical assistance can be availed. At the end of this chapter, some tips are given on how to prevent low blood pressure and complications related to it.

How to Diagnose and Evaluate?

In some patients, especially healthy and active ones, the symptoms of fainting, dizziness and fatigue are related to having low blood pressure most of the time. Others having these complications are often thought to have an event, such a heart attack.

The first step to diagnosing low blood pressure is to measure blood pressure both the standing and lying (supine) positions. The patients who suffer from symptomatic low blood pressure, they encounter a massive drop in blood pressure when they stand up. These patients may also develop symptoms of orthostatic hypotension and often the rate of heart beat reduces. The main purpose is to identify the root cause of low blood pressure. In some cases, the underlying reasons are readily apparent, such as sudden shock after applying X-ray dyes that contain iodine, or heavy loss of blood due to any trauma. Other times, the main reason can be found by performing some tests:

1. **Blood pressure test** – Your blood pressure is measured with a pressure-measuring gauge and an inflatable arm cuff. A blood pressure reading is measured in millimeters of mercury (mm Hg) and it is represented by two numbers. The first, or upper, limit determines the systolic pressure, that is, the pressure in your arteries when the heart beats. The second, or lower, limit determines the diastolic pressure, which is the pressure in the arteries between beats of the heart.

2. **CBC (Complete Blood Count)** – This test may identify either increased level of white blood cell due to severe infection, or anemia due to loss of blood.

3. **Blood electrolyte** – Measuring the electrolyte levels of blood may show kidney or renal failure, mineral shortage or dehydration and an excess amount of acid in the blood (acidosis).

4. **Urine and blood cultures** – These results will help in diagnosing bladder infections and septicemia, respectively.

5. **Cortisol measurement** – The levels can be measured to identify Addison's disease and adrenal insufficiency.

6. **Radiology studies** – Abdominal ultrasound, chest X-rays and computerized tomography (CT or CAT) scans are such radiological studies that can detect gallstone, heart failure, pneumonia, diverticulitis, and pancreatitis.

7. **Electrocardiograms** – EKG is used to detect pericarditis, abnormally rapid or slow heart beats and damage of heart muscles either from the previous event of heart attack or a decreased supply of blood to the heart muscle that still has not induced a heart attack.

8. **Holter monitor** – The readings can diagnose sporadic episodes of abnormal heart rhythms. A standard EKG test was done at the time your visit to your doctor's office may not reveal abnormal rhythms if this takes place intermittently. In that case, a Holter monitor is used that continuously monitor and record of the heart's rhythm for 24 hours. This recording is used to detect sporadic episodes of tachycardia or bradycardia.

9. **Patient-activated event recorder** – If the episodes of tachycardia or bradycardia do not take place frequently, then the intermittent episodes may not be captured by a recording of 24-hour Holter monitor. In this case, for 24 hours a patient can keep wearing a patient-activated recorder for 4 weeks. When the patient experiences the start of abnormal heart rhythm or possible symptoms related to low blood pressure, the patient can press the start button of the recorder. Later on, the doctor can analyze the recording to observe the abnormal episodes.

10. **Ultrasound examinations of leg vein and CT scans of chest** – Both these readings can identify pulmonary embolism and deep vein thrombosis.

11. **Echocardiograms** – These examine the motion and structure of the heart via ultrasound. The result can trace pericardial fluid due to pericarditis, rare tumors of the heart, diseases of the heart and extent of the damage to heart muscles caused due to heart attacks.

12. **Tilt-Table** – This test can assess suspected patients whether they have postural hypotension or syncope because of abnormal function of the autonomic nerves. During the test, the patient lies down on the observation table having an intravenous infusion administered and simultaneously the blood pressure and heart rate are monitored. Then for 15 minutes to 45 minutes, the table is tilted in an upright position. In every few minutes, blood pressure and rate of heart beat are recorded. The main aim of this test is to induce postural hypotension. Sometimes to reproduce postural hypotension, your doctor may intravenously administer epinephrine (Adrenalin, Isuprel).

13. **Valsalva maneuver** - This is a simple diagnosis designed for that part of the nervous system which controls the functions, such as the heartbeat and the constriction and expansion of the blood vessels. If something goes wrong with this mechanism of the nervous system, blood pressure issues may take place. During this test, all you have to do is to take a deep breath and then forcefully blow the air out through your lips. You need to do this several times. Your blood pressure and heart rate will be checked during the test.

14. **Stress test** – When the heart is beating fast and is working hard, then it is easier to identify the heart problems. This concept is being used in this test. During the stress test, doctors make you do exercise or give you medicines instead to make your heart beat faster and work harder. Then the heart test can be carried out. The heart tests may include echo, nuclear heart scanning and positron emission tomography (PET) scanning of your heart.

15. Echocardiography – In short, it is called "echo". It is a test which utilizes sound waves to create a motion image of the heart. The image displays the size and shape of your heart, as well as, how well your heart is functioning. There are many types of echo available and "stress echo" is one of them. Echo test is performed as part of the stress test. The stress echo is usually performed to investigate if you have reduced the flow of blood to your heart. If yes, then this is a sign that you have "coronary heart disease", also called "coronary artery disease".

Treatment of Low Blood Pressure

Healthy people with lower blood pressure reading without suffering from any symptom or organ damage usually do not require any treatment. Doctors should evaluate such kind of patients with possible low blood pressure signs. People who experience a sudden drop in their blood pressure than the normal reading must also get themselves checked by the doctors. At first, the doctors will advise the patients to perform some tests and other procedures to investigate the main reason behind the low blood pressure. Based on the result, appropriate treatments and remedies will be prescribed.

General advice to confront some symptoms of common types of low blood pressure are:

1. **Adjust medications by doctor's advice** – If the main reason for your low blood pressure is any medicine that you are taking at present, you should reduce the dose of the medicine or should completely stop taking it. Remember, you must not adjust the dose or stop taking it without consulting your doctor.

2. **Dehydration** – It is treated by consuming fluids and minerals or electrolytes. Mild dehydration without vomiting or nausea can be easily treated with the oral intake of electrolytes (minerals) and fluids. Intravenous electrolytes and fluids are given in hospital to treat patients with moderate to severe dehydration issue. If not treated, severe low blood pressure will make the patient go into shock.

3. **Blood loss** – Loss of blood can be taken care of by treating the cause of bleeding along with transfusion of blood and intravenous fluids. Whenever you suffer from severe and continuous bleeding, treat it immediately without delay.

4. **Septic shock** – This is a medical emergency and should be treated well with antibiotics and intravenous fluids.

5. **Blood pressure medications** – Doctors adjust, substitute or stop this type of drugs or diuretics if these are inducing low blood pressure.

6. **Bradycardia** – this may be caused due to any medication. The doctors may advise you to alter, reduce or stop taking it. An implantable pacemaker can be utilized to treat bradycardia which happens due to blocked heart or sick sinus syndrome.

7. **Tachycardia** – This condition is treated depending on the characteristics of tachycardia. The potential treatments of atrial fibrillation can be electrical cardioversion, oral medication, or pulmonary vein isolation (also known as, catheterization procedure). Implantable defibrillator or medicines can be used to control ventricular tachycardia.

8. **Deep vein thrombosis and pulmonary embolism** – These conditions can be treated with blood thinners, such as 'heparin' as an initial medication. After some time, oral 'warfarin' (Coumadin), or other oral drugs are used as substitutes instead of heparin.

9. **Pericardiocentesis** – This procedure can be used to extract pericardial fluid from pericarditis.

10. **Postprandial hypotension** – This health issue refers to low blood pressure occurring after meals. Ibuprofen (Motrin) or indomethacin (Indocin) may be used to treat this.

11. **Postural hypotension** – This low blood pressure can be treated by changing diet such as consuming increasing amount of salt and water, drinking more caffeinated beverages (as caffeine as the ability to narrow down blood vessels), administrating compression stocking to constrict the leg veins and decrease the collection of blood in the leg veins, and for some patients the usage of a medicine called "midodrine" (ProAmatine). Midodrine has some problems. When this medicine raises the blood pressure in the upright position, the supine blood pressure becomes very high. This elevates the risk of getting strokes. According to the Mayo Clinic researchers, there is a medicine that is used to treat weakness in muscles in "myasthenia gravis" known as "pyridostigmine" (Mestinon), which does not raise supine blood pressure but increases upright blood pressure. An anticholinesterase medication called "pyridostigmine" acts on the autonomic nervous system, particularly when a person is in stand up position. Increased frequency of bowel movements or minor abdominal cramping is some of the side-effects that are seen in this situation.

12. **Vasovagal syncope** – This condition can be treated with many types of medicines including beta-blockers, such as propranolol (Inderal, Inderal LA) and also selective serotonin reuptake inhibitors such as paroxetine (Paxil), sertraline (Zoloft), citalopram (Celexa), fluoxetine (Prozac), escitalopram oxalate (Lexapro), and fluvoxamine (Luvox). Another drug name Fludrocortisone (Florinef) can also be used to treat vasovagal syncope. This medicine makes your kidneys retain water in order to prevent dehydration. Furthermore, a pacemaker can also be an alternative when drug therapy fails to work on a patient.

13. **Herbal treatment** – Although natural remedy has not been yet proven to be effective in treating low blood pressure, but some herbs, like rosemary, aniseed, pepper, ginger and cinnamon, are reported by people to be good in increasing blood pressure. Never ingest any herbs without consulting your doctor, or else incorrect dosage or the herb itself can cause a reaction in your body.

Prevention of Low Blood Pressure

Hardly ever is treatment required for simple symptoms of low blood pressure like giddiness while standing and sometimes there aren't even symptoms to worry about.

Doctors typically strike at the heart of normal day-to-day health problems as a treatment for the cause of any symptom of low blood pressure such as diabetes, hypothyroidism or history of heart failure rather than fixating on low blood pressure in a whole.

Cures for episodes of low blood pressure from medicine normally range from changing the dose of the medication itself or just outright discontinuing it completely.

In such a case where the cause of low pressure is in doubt or if even a cure doesn't exist reducing signs and symptoms by increasing blood pressure is the go-to solution. It is all subject to the degree of low blood pressure, your health and age but you can do this in a number of ways, namely:

- **Use more salt.** Assimilating more salt into the body is a good thing for people with low blood pressure. The average person is usually told against including excess salt in their daily diet by nutrition experts as it increases blood pressure substantially.

  It's important to consult with your doctor before increasing daily salt intake because excess sodium can lead to heart failure, especially in older adults.

- **Drink more water.** Almost every human being is aided from drinking clean water but this is two-fold in the case of those suffering from low blood pressure.

  Fluids help avert dehydration and increase blood quantity which in turn treats hypotension.

- **Wear compression stockings.** Elastic coverings that are generally used to relieve the pain and swelling of varicose veins may help reduce the pooling of blood in your legs.

- **Medications.** Orthostatic hypotension, otherwise low blood pressure from standing up can be treated by one or more medications used in tandem with each other or separately.

  The drug fludrocortisone is habitually used to cure or treat this form of low blood pressure as it boosts your blood volume, which in turn raises blood pressure.

  The drug midodrine (Orvaten) has been commonly utilized by doctors to raise standing blood pressure levels in people with chronic orthostatic hypotension. It restricts the ability of your blood vessels to expand, which raises blood pressure.

You can take steps to help diminish or even prevent symptoms conditional on the reason for your low blood pressure. Recommendations include:

- **Drink more water, less alcohol.** Even if drunk sparingly, alcohol can be dehydrating and can lower blood pressure while water increases blood volume by hydrating the body cells.

- **Follow a healthy diet.** By including a diverse range of foods like vegetables, fruits, and whole grains, and fish and lean chicken, you can get all the nutrients you need for good health.

Add natural soy sauce or dry soup mixes to dressings and dips if your doctor insists you increase your salt intake but you aren't partial to food that may be a tad salty.

- **Go slowly when changing body positions.** By moving slowly from a prone to a standing position, you may be able to reduce the giddiness and nausea that arise from low blood pressure on standing.

Sleeping with the head of your bed slightly raised can treat your vertigo induced from gravity. Take breaths deeply for a few minutes before getting out of bed in the morning and then gently sit up before standing.

Cross your thighs in a scissors technique and squeeze if you begin to get symptoms while standing, or put one foot on the tip of a chair and lean as far forward as far as possible. These exercises encourage blood to flow from your legs to your heart.

- **Eat small, low-carb meals.** Eat small helpings several times a day and limit your daily intake of high-carbohydrate foods like rice, pasta, bread or potatoes to prevent blood pressure from dropping sharply after meals

Your doctor might recommend drinking tea or caffeinated coffee with meals to temporarily raise blood pressure, but because caffeine can cause additional problems, consult your doctor before drinking more caffeinated drinks.

Chapter 5- Some Extra Tips

Clinical Trial Tests

There are several associations that are completely committed to research focused on treating and preventing health complications regarding lung, heart and blood diseases and sleeping disorders. The national heart, Lung and Blood Institute (NHLBI) are one of them.

The studies supported by NHLBI have helped in the advancement in medical care and knowledge. Most of the time, these advancements depend on whether the volunteers are willing to take part in the clinical trials or not.

The mechanism of the clinical trials is based on experimenting with latest ways to prevent, diagnose, or do a treatment of various complications and diseases. For instance, latest treatments for a particular disease or health complication, such as medical devices, surgeries, drugs or methods, are all experimented on volunteers who have the same health condition. The test results show whether the new treatment or medicine is effective and safe to use for humans and then it is decided to launch in the market to be available for other people.

One of the advantages of taking part in clinical trials is that you can have easy access to latest treatments before these are even available widespread. In addition, you will have the medical support of a team of health care providers, who will closely observe your health condition. Even if you do not get much benefit from these clinical trials, still you will be able to gather enough information about the illness to guide others and add on to the information bank.

You might be thinking that taking clinical trials will be like being the experimental guinea pig to with which anything can happen, mostly bad consequences. Well, it is not true at all. If you take part in the clinical trials as a volunteer, the experts will explain you in details about the research and experiment they are about to do. They will also inform you about the tests and treatments you are going to receive and also the benefits and the possible side effects that might be associated with the procedure. If you have any query or question, you can ask the experts and verify everything about the research and the required procedures. This process is known as "informed consent".

After knowing all these information, if you agree to take part in the clinical trial, then you will be given a form of consent to sign. This is not a contractual form. You will have the liberty to quit from the research for any kind of reason and at any time. In addition, you can be acknowledged about the new findings and risk factors that may arise during the trial.

Conclusion

Whether it is for a minute or two or it is stretched out for hours on end, the effects of low blood pressure are real and tangible and affect many of all around us. To feel better you just have to use some of the day-to-day techniques and implement certain mentioned diets into breakfast, lunch and dinner. You don't need to be as systematic as a computer or as punctual as a clock, trying is the first step and is the one that really matters. If you don't give it a shot how will you know if it works or not? You may find it hard to eat fare that is a tad salty, but drinking water and eating low-carb meals will help tremendously to cure your hypotension. And if salt is a major problem, just add a dash of salt to everyday meals as no one expects you sprinkle bucket loads into the dish! These small steps may seem inconsequential but they go the distance to help alleviate your lightheadedness. Soon your blood pressure will stabilize, your body will work like a well-oiled machine, and vertigo from standing will be a thing of the past.

We really care about Your opinion on the book. Please write a review or just rate it on Amazon.com. Thank You!

www.ingramcontent.com/pod-product-compliance
Lightning Source LLC
Chambersburg PA
CBHW071300280526
45788CB00004B/1789